Prepare Me To

Train

Using anime for proper mindset, weight-training, and nutrition

Copyright © 2024 by Antonio J. Savage

Prepare Me To Train

Using anime for proper mindset, weight-training, and nutrition

Antonio J. Savage

Dedication

This book is dedicated to my mother Arleen, for letting me watch all the anime I wanted,

taking me to Karate classes, supporting at Football games, and showing me how to

survive.

We've been through a lot together, and I appreciate you for supporting me in my business

and in all that I showed interest in over the years.

Thank you for providing the atmosphere for me to grow and develop into a man of

creativity.

Contents

Dedication 4

Introduction 6

Dragon ball 9

Pokémon 15

Samurai Jack 23

Vitamins and Supplements 29

Training Concepts 37

Bonus 41

References 43

Acknowledgement 46

Introduction

Training concepts are what we are talking about here that can literally be used for every aspect of getting better in life. When I say the concept of training, I'm talking about getting your mind prepared and ready to train. We'll talk more at the end about preparing yourself for training.

Training is really just creating a habit. A habit is a pathway of doing things.

When you do something over and over, you're constructing a street, then a road, then a highway of pathways in your brain. Adapting to the change of our habits is what we perceive as growth, development, and results. When we create new habits, we create new lifestyles. Those habits come from thoughts or good ideas. Those thoughts come from outside sources, normally, and come through the five senses of experience. One big avenue for learning new habits, of which is often overlooked or not spoken of often, is anime.

I was raised by Bloodsport 1 & 2, Dragon Ball, Pokémon, Digimon, The Drunken Master, The Last Dragon, Samurai Jack, and the like. From all of them, I learned perseverance, dedication, determination, grit, anything is possible, tenacity, discipline, and fight. Being a millennial, my generation invested much time into television, but the message was mostly educational.

- The first season of Crashbox premiered on HBO Family on February 1, 1999.
- Bill Nye the Science Guy aired from September 10, 1993 to June 20, 1998, hosted by William "Bill" Nye and produced by Buena Vista Television.
- The Magic School Bus --original TV series-- was broadcast on PBS from 1994 until 1997.
- Blue's Clues premiered in the U.S. on September 8, 1996.
- Arthur began airing on October 7, 1996.

All these shows were very educational and I learned quite a bit, because they were interesting. I'm not going to put down any shows that are out for education today, but I do appreciate the ones that I've mentioned here. There were also out of the box thinking movies:

- The Matrix opened in theaters in the United States on March 31, 1999.
- Enemy of the State was released on November 20, 1998.
- Malcolm X was distributed by Warner Bros. and released in the United States on November 18, 1992.

All these movies were about waking up to the reality of betrayal and seeking the truth.

Now, I'm a man of faith. I believe in God wholeheartedly and I believe that he helped my mother raise me, being that my father wasn't there, for the most part, except a few summers and here and there's. I relate very closely with the movie 'Boyz In The Hood' - another very educational movie - in that my parents weren't together, yet they played their part in my life. I love, honor, and respect my father for being my father and for continuing to be in my life; and for the things that I learned watching him.

I still attribute the four-mentioned shows and movies as a big part of my upbringing, and I'll spend the rest of the time gifted to us together in sharing why that is, with three animes that taught me lessons for life I will never forget.

Dragon Ball

The first time I saw Dragon Ball, I was six years old. It was 'The Garlic Jr. Saga.' I remember seeing Piccolo's big green arms on the big screen TV, and he and Krillin fighting Gohan just to throw Garlic Jr. off, making him think that both he and Krillin were under his spell and they were fighting to kill the young boy, but then suddenly turning on him to fight alongside Gohan. Gohan, who eventually defeated Garlic for the second time by throwing him into the Dead zone for all eternity, was glad he still had friends on his side even though he could've beat them.

Since then, I have been hooked on Dragon Ball and all of its franchises, including Dragon Ball, Dragon Ball Z, the latest Dragon Ball Super and even a little of Dragon Ball GT. The biggest influence from the anime for me has got to be the training. Master Roshi, an old frail-looking guy, showed Goku and Krillin how to push past human limits with hard work.

In training, you'll come across walls that you will hit and you have to break through those walls. The sweat equity these boys learned made them unstoppable in the ring and in life. Master Roshi taught Goku and Krillin that if they just push past all human limits, no one would be able to give them a hard time.

It was because of DragonBall and DragonBall Z that I began training in fitness and martial arts. It even had a big role in my decision in 2011 to become a personal trainer. It's currently 2024 and though I've trained others on and off since 2011, I've always been a trainer and a mentor at heart. On my mother's side of the family, I am the youngest of three siblings. Both of my siblings are at least eight years older than me. However, my mom recalled to me a time when my siblings were arguing over something. I had gotten in-between them and started counseling them on loving each other as brother and sister and not fighting. They all looked at me, looked at each other and started laughing at the audacity, the cuteness and the boldness of this young man to take leadership out of all of them and guide the way.

Later, when I married my wife Priscilla, I helped her go from 134 lbs to (170 - 175) lbs at 5 ft 7. She was a stick figure when we met and now she's a brick house. That means she's fine. She's stronger, she's healthier and has the right meat - or lean muscle mass, in the right places, to say the least. Some people have a different goal, but hers is actually to gain more and I'm going to train her on doing it the healthy way.

Master Roshi gave me one of my biggest methods for training using weights. I started weight-training at the age of six by the way. Roshi not only introduced weight-training, but he showed how you could get faster and stronger by doing hard work while using the weights to increase the resistance. Resistance can be seen as a bad thing, but it's actually very necessary in the development of strength and muscles, as well as getting better at handling the many challenges life throws at us.

I was also very interested in the weighted clothing idea a little later in the series where Goku took off 100 kgs when he took off his shirt, boots, and wrist bands in the 23rd Tenkaichi

Budokai martial arts tournament, which he ended up winning. I believe that this type of training can be realistic if practiced with care.

In a blog post by Mark Heidelberger, he mentions that Terry Downey, a physical therapist at Harvard-affiliated Spaulding Rehabilitation Network says it's not a good idea to use wearable ankle weights while you're walking or during an aerobics workout, because they force you to use your quadriceps (the muscles in the fronts of the thighs) and not your hamstrings (in the backs of the thighs). "That causes a muscle imbalance." (Heidelberger, n.d.). This would make your quadriceps work more than your hamstrings which can lead to injuries in your knees, hips, and back. Downey also warns against weighted wristbands and vests on the bases of imbalances occurring.

The key takeaways from Downey's concerns are, "imbalances." Now imbalances occur when you tighten, or contract a muscle group too often without tightening or contracting the opposite or eccentric muscle group. Each muscle group can contract concentrically or eccentrically and they take turns when they are in the same area of the body. Example: The muscle in front of your tibialis anterior (this is the front of your lower leg) contracts concentrically when you release your foot from the gas pedal and from the brake pedal of your vehicle. Your gastrocnemius muscle or calf muscle, contracts concentrically when you press down on the pedal. Both of these muscles work at the same time but not in concentric contraction. When you press down on the pedal, your gastrocnemius muscle contracts concentrically while your tibialis anterior muscle contracts eccentrically; and when you release from the pedal, the opposite effect happens.

Imbalances are real, however, have you stopped to consider how we move throughout the day? Wouldn't we always be creating imbalances, as we do not evenly move so that every muscle and joint receives an even proportion of resistance?

Think about the realities of this when you gain weight. You have more weight on you, now should there be a concern for imbalances? Maybe in hormonal imbalances, but not necessarily in movement. The case for imbalances comes into play when you overuse or overwork a group of muscles and joints. An example of this is Brake Press Operators. These labor workers are often tasked with work that requires them to consistently lift heavy metals to bend them to different angles, sometimes in very awkward positions of which they often have hundreds of parts to bend. Shoulders like that become imbalanced and may lead to a shorter range of motion, pain or even numbness.

For the case of weighted vests, wrists and ankles, I propose using such equipment only if you understand the kinesiology of the body and know how to stretch. Using a group of muscles too often can bring an imbalance in tightness if you don't stretch or know how to stretch the right muscles. There is Dynamic stretching, Ballistic stretching, and Static stretching. That is something that could've been explored more in the Dragon Ball franchise for individuals wanting to train like the characters in the story. I often tell people who ask me for fitness advice,

"Stretching is like oil, if you don't use it, you will become like a tin man." I also say, "If you don't stretch, you'll turn into an old man/woman quickly."

Goku and Krillin both already had training in martial arts. They actually had mad skills at the ages of 12 and 13, yet they recognized that they could benefit many times faster with having a mentor who's been where they wanted to be and who could help them get there. To be technical, Roshi didn't teach them how to *fight*. He taught them how to *train*. He did this with everyday things like swimming, delivering milk, and labor construction work. These may seem like normal things, but they were all intensified. Swimming in a lake of shark-infested water and holding a case of milk straight in front of you for miles and miles is one thing, but as stated before, heavy boulders were put on their backs! Their training was not only physical, but mental as well with math and other subjects. Roshi conditioned Goku and Krillin so much that they were able to knock down big, bulky men with so much as a finger tap, and their minds were sharp enough to where they could come up with their own strategies on outsmarting their opponents.

Later on, in Dragon Ball Z, the sequel to Dragon Ball, we see Gohan - Goku's son - and Krillin doing mind-training. They are telepathically sparing with each other. We see this again in Dragon Ball Super when Freeza is brought back to the living world for one day, and he mentions that he has been mentally training the entire time he was in Earth's hell. Now there is a lot of legitimacy in this style of training - not the coming back from the dead for a day training, but mind training.

For one, our brains are like computers. We can literally program our minds to believe whatever we want. The downfall to this is, so can everyone else. This is why we must guard our mind from both negative people and well-meaning individuals who are negative with their beliefs or who don't believe that you can achieve what you want to achieve. Protect it at all costs! This is where possibilities are allowed and the impossible is made possible.

Scientifically speaking, the neurons in your brain are structured like roads. Your experience is what has constructed those roads. If you want to train for a specific purpose that may seem out of your reach currently, it's time for construction. You construct by meditating on what you want. Meditation is not being empty-minded, it is actually focusing on what you want or just focusing on something. In your case it's a desired result.

Words are powerful. This is talked about in many books and audios from Shad Helmstetter where he mentions neuroplasticity. Self-talk is also used by athletes and those looking to lose weight (Helmstetter & Schwartz, 1996). Studies have shown that athletes who utilize positive self-talk during competition experience improved performance, confidence, focus, and emotional regulation. This mindset of attitude leads to overcoming challenges and outperforming others who don't use self-talk. Shad speaks on self-talk as his key to losing unwanted weight in an audio called 'The Science Behind Self-talk' and even has a book called 'Self-talk For Weight Loss.'

It's very interesting to see shows like Dragon Ball articulate styles of training that are used today. There are many more concepts to take from the franchise, but these are three key concepts talked about here:
- Mentorship
- Mind-training
- Weight-training

Watching Goku and Krillin train as young boys, having a master or teacher guiding them along their journeys had the biggest impact on me; and I am very appreciative of the work of original Author Akira Toriyama for bringing such art, philosophy and purpose to my life. Much respect for him and his family, and may he rest in honor and peace.

Pokémon

So I've talked about overtraining muscles, and there's no other system that has taught me this lesson but Pokémon. Now, I'm not as fanatical about Pokémon as I am about Dragon Ball, but when I was coming up, Gameboy Advance had a huge pull on me. I literally stayed up playing during the entire day; and I would play throughout the entire night until it was day again and still wanted to keep going. If it wasn't for silly things like school and batteries dying, I probably wouldn't stop. Looking back, I guess it could've been seen as an addiction, but it definitely held my attention. I was so fascinated by the world created in my game that I basically lived vicariously through the characters - or rather through the trainer I played as. I even played Dragon Ball Z on the Gameboy, but nothing was as interesting to me as Pokémon.

What interested me the most wasn't catching the most Pokémon, no. It was training them and battling with others. However, my inner self would sort of chide me when I played too much. That inner voice was saying, "You're training your Pokémon to get stronger and better, but you're not training yourself." I think that was a little bit of Dragon Ball Z in my consciousness holding me accountable. I calmed down a bit on playing so often after that conversation.

I learned quite a lot from Pokémon. Before learning about photosynthesis in school, I had already learned from training my grass-type Pokémon and looking up some of the words I had to read while playing the game. I learned the weaknesses and strengths of elements based on the weaknesses and strengths of the types of Pokémon. At this present moment, I'm thinking about the creators of Pokémon and the game for it as utter geniuses! That was a fun way to train my mind for success. It was also a fun way of retaining what I learned, because I would have to if I was going to win battles against other trainers who knew their stuff.

As I mentioned at the beginning of this chapter, one of the lessons I learned from playing Pokémon was about overuse. Here's a scene for explanation: Let's say you're playing Pokémon X game on a Gameboy PSP and you come across a very strong trainer with Pokémon who are the same type as yours. Their attacks don't really hurt much but they still have to use the moves they know. There are only four moves Pokémon can use and each move tells you how many times you can use that move. Once your moves go down to zero, your Pokémon has no use but to struggle because they've used all their moves too many times. In struggling, they give damage to the other Pokémon, but they also damage themselves a little. That's exactly how it is when you overuse your muscles to the point they are too tight and are imbalanced. Common sense about overuse is seen in moderations.

Now, in the game, when your Pokémon uses up all of their moves, you can either give them an item called Ether - which replenishes their ability to do their moves, or you can take them to a Pokémon Center. In other words, a hospital, and they'll be fully healed and able to use their moves again. This isn't a book on how to play Pokémon, yet it is a cross reference to our own bodies' abilities to use and overuse our muscles. I only wish we had something as simple as Ether to replenish our ability to move like we used to before overusing and imbalancing our muscles. The fact that the Pokémon need to go to the hospital to get their ability to move again shows how serious overuse is. What we can do instead of going to the hospital is to prevent overuse by proper movement, much stretching, vitamins and supplements, and much, much rest.

Pokémon, as you know, is a fantasy idea, though it may have many lessons that are real. One of the fantasies which many wish were real is what's called Rare Candy. This item levels a Pokémon up without them having to train. If this was a real thing, many would use it as a top dollar exchange. In a way, more money can give you a higher status. So can the invention of some new technology. However, those things are mostly gained over time. Fast money is lost or spent fast. Slow money is cherished, invested, and grows overtime.

If there was a Rare Candy in the real world, it would spoil the stomach and give no real nutrients. Getting something for nothing takes away the process of development that comes only through the resistance of the challenge. You learn nothing. You don't experience the pain which takes away the ability and capacity of experiencing the joy. It's just like aging with no new knowledge or wisdom. You're not more mature, you're just older at the same level of ignorance.

There is one thing I took advantage of in the game of Pokémon. Well, when I first started playing Pokémon on Gameboy Advance, it was second generation. And I had almost all of the games, starting with Pokémon Crystal, then Gold - The Kanto region, for those Pokémon Vets out there. This is important to note, because you couldn't run like you could in the later generations of the game - by later generations, I mean later versions. This means it took time to travel to each phase of the game. That's one of the reasons I would stay up all night playing until the batteries died. Then I'd scramble for more! That being said, it took time to level up. Of course, if you found a Rare Candy that saved you a lot of time.

Each city that you traveled to normally had a Gym where you could earn badges by defeating the Gym Leaders, of which were always about five to ten levels stronger than the last Gym Leaders in the previous city. Traveling from one city to the next, you'd go through roads and paths that connected the cities. During these travels, there are other trainers who will challenge you to a battle. There are also patches of grass that if you go into, you can be met with wild Pokémon that you can either catch, battle, or flee from. Realizing this, I decided to stay in the patches of grass to battle Pokémon over and over again until my Pokémon reached a level that would allow me to use one move and defeat other Pokémon. This way, whenever I finally went to battle the Gym Leaders, I could use one Pokémon for each trainer instead of risking an 'even battle' that could lead to overuse of moves and fainting of Pokémon from being too damaged. A great example I can remember is training one of my Pokémon to level 30, letting it evolve and then going to battle Gym Leaders whose highest level Pokémon was 15.

Now this was a great lesson! I learned to hone my skills and abilities and to level up to be ready for the next challenge life threw at me. You can do this as well. Just ask yourself a few questions:

- What are my goals?
- What challenges may come up in the pursuit of my goals?
- How can I level up before I encounter these challenges?

Before I went to high school, I heard many rumors and even saw movies and TV shows that depicted things like "Freshman Friday," where seniors would take a freshman and give him what's known as a swirly. A swirly is when you get your head dipped in a toilet and are sort of drowned a bit until you manage to flush the toilet and breathe. In my last year of Middle School, I contemplated this and decided to take matters into my own hands.

No, I did not think about bringing artillery to the school to protect myself, nor did I come up with a tattle tell system. I simply trained. I trained my butt off getting ready for whatever was to come and whoever wanted to try something. Thankfully, my training paid off and nobody messed with me. I was the buff kid at school.

I remember when my mother and I had just moved to San Diego and we were struggling. We lived in a women's shelter for a little while before we eventually got an apartment. While we were at the shelter, there were some rules. A child could not go anywhere without their mother, and that included being able to come into the shelter without their mother. I was 15 at the time, and my mother worked second shift as a security officer downtown, so I often had to wait at a restaurant and would meet her there so that we could both go into the shelter together as she would get off work by 10pm. Even though I was 15, the age limit for a "child" was 17. So I couldn't even go to the restroom without my mom, and it was lights out by about 9pm. Oh yeah, and we shared a room with two beds. It was like we were on lockdown. But this, I took advantage of.

From my training in Pokémon, I saw this as an opportunity to level up and embrace the prison-like scene. I took it upon myself to institutionalize myself in getting better by honing my mind. I would think of controversial conversations and attacking comments and I would come up with responses. My mom and I would challenge each other on the meaning of Scripture and we sharpened each other in debates as iron sharpens iron. I became extremely sharp and prepared, surprising all who I spoke with. This allowed me to jump from regular class studies to all AP classes. I was also being considered for skipping a grade, until I started associating with my peers who were apathetic to a degree I thought was only reserved for special education elementary. This, I recognized and was disgusted by, because I had grown to love wisdom. I also worked so hard to get to where I was, as I had leveled up from special education classes myself.

Here's how I recognized what was going on. In the Women's shelter, we were required to go to therapy. I felt like I had no need for it and believed strongly that I could actually help the therapist trying to "reach" me. Our first couple of sessions, I impressed her tremendously. I'm not reading my own press clippings, she told me this. But in the very last session, I felt dumbfounded and explained that she caught me off guard. What has really happened, was that my social life was becoming a hindrance to my grasp on intelligence. I had not yet figured out how to balance social life with my personal development. I was able to level up in my personal development and even had someone to sharpen my mind further with challenging my thoughts, but learning how to blend a holistic approach to growth was lacking.

You see, in the game of Pokémon, when you level the Pokémon up, everything levels up. Strength. Speed. Accuracy. Defense. Not so in real life. We are complex creatures. God has made us the pinnacle of creation; and having the ability to create is a strong reason why. But we also have many states that we can level up in. We have Science, History, Philosophy, Health, Relationships, Spirituality, Inventions, etc. But I believe there are things we can level up in that we haven't even tapped into yet! I guess you can technically put all human study in the category of Science, but here's how I see it:

Scientists are little children everyday discovering what their Father (God) has already created.

Satoshi Tajiri is the creator of the Pokémon franchise, and again, I say, what a genius, to create such an educational and fun way of learning. Tajiri got his concept of Pokémon from his childhood hobby of collecting bugs (Ameridisability, 2018). This is true entrepreneurship. Training at its best is learning lessons as you are on the field of battle. You can learn away from the battle, but some things are only learned on the field.

One of my mentors always says, "Many things are taught, but some of the most important things can only be caught."

- What can we catch in battle?

1. Always level up before battles come to you. In other words, learn to swim before you're thrown in; and dig your well before you're thirsty.

2. Battle strengths against weaknesses.

3. Avoid overusing or overworking your muscles, your hobbies, your gaming, your visits with friends and family or anything else that should be in moderation.

Samurai Jack

Samurai Jack was almost on par with Dragon Ball for me. This is a character that was a hero and the last hope of his village to stop the evil wizard Aku from taking over and ruling the world. Jack has a sword that could cut through anything, given to him from his ancestors, and he is extremely skilled with it. He almost completely defeats Aku, but Aku throws Jack into the future where Aku already rules the world and Jack has to both adapt to the future and fight off all of the assassins sent by Aku to kill him.

There were a few scenes in this epic, exciting and futuristic show that really grasped my attention in terms of training that I appreciated from creator Genndy Tartakovsky. Season 2: episode 14, which aired on March 1, 2002 is when Jack learned how to "jump good." The episode starts out with Jack being teased by Aku who simply outsized Jack by growing taller or turning into a bat-like creature. Jack, used to ground fights, is treated as a younger, shorter brother trying desperately to reach Aku to connect an attack, in vain. Jack then goes off to a land where beast-like characters show him how to "jump good." Jack didn't just see them jump good and start jumping good, he had to train to jump good like them.

The main thing they used in Jack's training is oversized boulders - which is basically the same method of training Master Roshi incorporated with his training. After a time of living like the beasts live, jumping from tree to tree and running everywhere, Jack is allowed to release the giant boulder from his back and jumps so high he can give the impression that he is flying, and this is with very little effort. Jack, at the end of the episode then confronts Aku who laughs at Jack and tries to embarrass him again with being just out of his reach in their fight, but Jack surprises Aku by reaching him easily. Aku cries out, "You can fly?!!" And Jack says, "no, Jump Good!" And the episode ends.

MasterClass Instructor, Joe Holder, suggests that Walking with weights intensifies the workout to increase calorie burn and muscle toning. Depending on your fitness goals and where you place the added weight, you can activate your upper body or further challenge your lower-body muscles during your walking workout (MasterClass, 2021).

I actually tested the training method of Roshi and Jack on myself for a month. For an entire month, I wore 20 lbs ankle weights on each of my legs. During this time, I didn't have a vehicle and I didn't have transportation, but I did attend an in-person college in Georgia. I also went to the library almost everyday to do my work while using their wifi. How did I get around? I walked - with my ankle weights on the entire time. The only time I took them off was to wash up. I often practiced Capoeira (an African-Brazilian martial art that was used by African slaves to free themselves from their Brazilian slave masters) with them during this time as well, which required much footwork.

After a month of ankle weights, I finally took them off and felt just like Jack. Well, the feeling was mostly in my legs. I noticed as I walked to my different destinations that a simple step forward was so light. My legs literally felt like feathers. I would move my leg forward and it would swing almost all the way up to my face! Walking was extremely fun and light. I also felt like Goku did in the 23rd tournament after taking off his weighted clothing. He literally created a twister storm throwing punches and kicks. I could kick and flip with no problem at all. Now, I did train in martial arts with this weight on me, but for the most part, I went through my regular day. Think about the military training and how much Rangers must carry with them. No imbalances heard of there. I'm sure they understand the feeling after taking such a load off.

Another episode of Jack showed me great mind training. Jack and the Three Blind Archers is the seventh episode of the first season of Samurai Jack. Jack must get past three powerful archers to reach a wish-granting well. He is brutally defeated and realizes that he needs to use a different method.
He needs to fight on their level. He needs to use his other senses and not rely so much on his eyesight.

He went to be alone and blindfolded himself. Abandoning his sense of sight, Jack was about to focus on everything around him, The deer scratching the snow to find grass to eat, The birds fluttering their wings, The melting of the ice creating a puddle of water. Being able to focus, Jack went back and out-performed the blind archers.

This is big training right here. There is a famous quote by Blaise Pascal that goes like this, "All of humanity's problems stem from man's inability to sit quietly in a room alone." When you type this quote in Google search, AI says it's often due to feelings of anxiety, boredom, or the inability to manage the silence.

I believe this quote to be true most of the time. However, if a person is often alone, they tend to learn how to first cope with solitude and later prefer it. Whatever the case, Jack was able to consecrate his mind to focus. There are two things going on here. Firstly, Jack reflects what happened and he pays attention to the details of his failure. Secondly, Jack focuses on leveling up specifically in his keen awareness. He's already fast. He's already accurate. It was his attention that was lacking. When Jack blinded himself, he simply noticed his surroundings. He recognized that the semantic noise was actually his eyesight. The Archers, being blind with no semantics, knew where everything was. Jack was a newbie.

This often happens in our lives, especially in chasing a goal. We come across challenges that are in beast mode compared to our level of competency and we fail to rise to the new high standard of the challenge. Most will give up, some will try again and few will level up to overcome. Which one are you?

No matter who you are, you can level up to overcome. Recognize where you're incompetent.

Raise your abilities in that area and try again.

Think about this, absolutely everyone on earth is born a winner. How is that? Well, first off, we've all won the race to be born! Have you stopped to consider how difficult that was? How many challenges we overcame, how many other potentials could've gotten to the finish line before us?

In the process of conception, there are over three million sperms (that's you and me) that race to fertilize one egg, and as soon as that egg is fertilized, there's a burst of light that occurs! (National Institutes of Health, 2011).

Wow! Now that's perspective.

One of my mentors told me, "Life is 50% attitude. And the other half, is attitude."

You'll gain confidence from building your abilities. Having confidence is almost winning the entire battle. Of course, you also need effort to complete the task. I will put it this way: just as fitness is said to be 80% diet and 20% workouts, just as football is 80% strategy/plan and 20% work, so winning is 80% confidence and 20% effort. If you're familiar with the 80/20 rule, isn't it interesting to realize the different aspects of our lives it can be applied to?

The 80% fail to rise and adapt to the rushing standards of life challenges constantly outstretching your reach. Only the 20% train and sharpen and hone their craft of being, so that they may overcome to become better.

- Are you a part of the 80% or the 20%?

Vitamins and Supplements

This is a big subject in the health and wellness world, as well as the training world; and there's a good reason for it. In most cases, these products really aid you in your training. Let's dig into it.

The body needs six essential nutrients to function well, and they are:

Carbohydrates, Proteins, Fats, Vitamins, Minerals, and Water

You can get this from your diet.

Here is a five color code cheat sheet for you to easily remember through your diet what foods to eat to obtain your essential nutrients:

Green = Cellular Health

Yellow/Orange = Eye Health

Purple = Brain Health

Red = Blood Health

White = Bone Health

From these colorful foods, the body can obtain the essential nutrients it needs. Does your plate have all of these colors each day? If not, you may want to consider filing in the color gaps. This is where vitamins and supplements come in.

Your body needs vitamins in order to function properly. Vitamins are organic molecules that are essential to an organism in small quantities for proper metabolic function ("Vitamin," n.d.). The metabolism is what regulates the process of food turning into energy in your body. The more you exercise, the higher your metabolism. The more you're stagnant, the lower your metabolism. Here are 13 essential vitamins:

Vitamins A, B vitamins (Thiamine, Riboflavin, Niacin, Pantothenic acid, Biotin, B6, B12, and Folate), C, D, E and K.

There are vitamins that we need that the body naturally produces and there are vitamins that the body does not produce. The vitamins that our body produces are vitamins D and K, and it can synthesize niacin from the amino acid tryptophan (Carpenter et al., 2024). Here are the vitamins that you can only get from food:

Thiamine (vitamin B1), Riboflavin (vitamin B2), Pantothenic acid (vitamin B5), Biotin, vitamin B6, vitamin B9 (Folate), vitamin B12 (Cobalamin), vitamin C.

That's eight vitamins that the body needs and can't produce on its own! Being that we cannot produce these vitamins in the body, we must obtain them through diet or through supplements.

If you've seen Dragon Ball Super, you'll know that both characters, Vegeta and Goku are big eaters. They will eat and eat and eat. It's no wonder they are the main characters in the story saving the day from utter destruction, they have the most energy, or *should* at least from all of their intake. They probably have three times the daily recommendation of nutrients, which may not be that good, if you want to try and eat like them. The idea of eating more to be able to produce more effort is solid and legit, because food is absorbed and turned into energy, simply put. This goes into metabolism that I mentioned earlier. However, if you're not as active as Goku and Vegeta, you should stick with the daily recommended intake, otherwise, you will end up looking like Majin Buu. If you don't know who that is, look him up.

Just what is this Daily Recommended Intake? It actually originated from the RDA or Recommended Dietary Allowance.

The first edition of the Recommended Dietary Allowances (RDAs) was published in 1943 during World War II with the objective of "providing standards to serve as a goal for good nutrition." It defined, in "accordance with newer information, the recommended daily allowances for the various dietary essentials for people of different ages" (NRC, 1943). The origin of the RDAs has been described in detail by the chairman of the first Committee on Recommended Dietary Allowances (National Research Council, 1989).

Let's take a look at the RDA for fruits and vegetables:

- The daily recommended fruit intake for adults is 1.5 - 2 cups daily, and for vegetables it's 2 - 3 cups daily (Lee et al., 2022).

Are you getting the daily recommended fruits and veggies? I don't know about you, but I don't meet that recommendation daily. That is why I supplement with the best products on the market, in my opinion. Being that I have a background in health and wellness, naturally, I'm very picky about what I put into my body. The products that I use are NSF Certified.

NSF is the only independent, third-party testing organization that offers true testing of dietary supplements on their own laboratories to verify that products are safe and high quality by meeting industry standards of which is also tested for banned substances. They conduct annual audits and periodically retest certified products to ensure they continue to meet the organization's rigorous standards (National Sanitation Foundation, n.d.). NSF also insures:

- The product's contents match the label

- The product is free of contaminants like heavy metals, pesticides, and herbicides

- The product follows good manufacturing practices (GMPs)

Oh, and the daily recommended fruit intake for kids is 1.5 - 2.5 daily and 1 - 3 cups for vegetables (Mayo Clinic, n.d.). Are your kids getting the recommended fruits and veggies? There's great news for you - there are actually a lot of NSF Certified supplements for kids of all ages and in many different forms. There are splats, drops, gummies, smoothies and more. I recommend you get some type of supplement that fills the gaps for you and the kids in your life, of which is NSF Certified, of course. Be sure to read till the end to benefit from an offer I'm giving to those who are interested in learning more about filling the gaps of nutrients through vitamins and supplements.

In Dragon Ball, there is a super supplement that's called, "senzu beans." These amazing supplements are able to cure a person from almost anything. They don't work on viruses - which is funny, because when you go to the doctors office to be seen about a cold, the doctor gives you antibiotics, but antibiotics don't work on viruses (Kern, 2023). But if you are near death, you will be fully healed with the "senzu beans." I wish we had such technology in the real world. These senzu beans also serve another purpose: they keep you full for an entire day. As a matter of fact, I think they keep you full for a few days, so you can eat them alone.

Do not make the mistake of only taking supplements and eating nothing else. Supplements are not intended to take the place of meals, they are to fill in the gaps. I repeat, we have not found a way to create senzu beans yet!

Dietary supplements add nutrients to your diet and are intended to lower the risk of health problems. They are available over-the-counter, online, or from direct distributors in a variety of forms, including pills, capsules, powders, liquids, and gummies.

Supplements can contain:

Vitamins, Minerals, Fiber, Amino Acids, Herbs or other Plants, and Enzymes.

Supplements are not drugs or medicine and are not meant to cure diseases. Supplements are intended to prevent diseases from happening rather than curing them. However, my wife and I have customers who have told us testimonies of speedy recoveries from diseases like COVID 19, Migraines and Headaches, and an older gentleman going from being bedridden, getting taken care of by his daughter to healthy and strong, living on his own!

It really does pay to fill in the gaps for the long run or for a long healthy life. You may think you're good without supplements and function fine, but after a while you'll start to notice a decline in functionality, especially after the age of 30. I don't wish it upon you, but it normally starts to make sense around that age, especially if you're not as active as you used to be. Trust me. Here are a few vitamins and minerals and the areas of health they help with:

Zinc - promotes skin health and slows down vision loss

Melatonin - helps with sleep

Folic acid - good for childbearing-age women

Omega-3 fatty acids - helps with heart

Calcium and vitamin D - helps with strong bones and prevents the loss of bone density

Vitamins A, C, and E - helps with eyes

Probiotics - helps with digestion and the immune system

In Pokémon, you're actually able to purchase nutrients from shops to give to your Pokémon and they'll become stronger in that area. For example, if you were to buy Calcium for a Pokémon and gave it to it, its special attack would increase. A special attack is a Pokémon's strengths, like sit-ups are some individuals' strengths while it is others' weaknesses. Pokémon is a strength against a weakness. If you gave the Pokémon Zinc, their special defense would increase. Special defense is defense against special attacks or attacks that target their weaknesses like water to fire - fire would strengthen its defense against water, or fire to ice - ice would strengthen its defense against fire. It's essentially strengthening your defense against crisis events like wars or pandemics.

Zinc for us in the real world helps the immune system by helping white blood cells fight off infections and viruses, and it helps for wound-healing and tissue repair. And of course, Calcium helps with strong bones, but did you know that Vitamin K is important for the regulation of Calcium? Calcium is directly affected by the amount of vitamin K in the body (Hu et al., 2021). That's food for thought.

Supplements are not approved by the FDA because they are not food and they are not drugs (U.S. Food & Drug Administration, 2023). Many don't know what the FDA is. It is an acronym for the Food & Drug Administration. Drugs or medication tend to have undesirable side effects when you take them, because they are actually chemicals that alter diseases. They can also alter the mind and lead to intoxication. Genetically, drugs can be dangerous with the wrong concoction. Be aware that drugs can actually give you mental disorders (Casagrande Tango, 2003).

Instead of FDA, you should look for supplements that are NSF Certified. Most drugs or medication have side effects due to the chemicals in them, yet the FDA still approves them to the public. Some supplements actually have side effects as well, which shows that you must do your research for over-the-counter supplements. This is why you want to choose supplements that are NSF Certified and organic. The supplements I use, on the other hand, do not have side effects because they are all NSF Certified, there's no chemicals and they have their own birthday certificate - meaning I have the ability to trace them all the way back to when the seed form was planted, until the time it was put into capsule form or any of the other forms. Remember that anything taken in excess is bad, but the proper dosage can yield various benefits.

Training Concepts

In ancient times, Nubia was known as the "Land of the Bow." Nubian hunters and warriors excelled as archers, and their weapon became a symbol for Nubia. "Land of the Bow" is the meaning of Ta-Seti, an ancient Egyptian term used to denote Nubia for thousands of years in antiquity. However, if we were to take the most accurate of archers from ancient times Nubia and put him in a competition against Nicholas James Vujicic, Nicholas would hit the bullseye first - if, that is, the Nubian was first blindfolded, spun around seven times to the right, then five times to the left. Why? Well, have you ever been blindfolded and spun around? Unless you know how to use Ultra Instinct, where your body moves and reacts on its own based on experience, you won't know where you are, let alone where the target is.

Want to know why I picked Nicholas as the challenger? Well, Nick may not be an archer, but he's a golfer, a swimmer, a skydiver, an actor, an acclaimed author, a musician, a motivational speaker, an Australian-American Christian Evangelist and a father of four. Seems like a cool enough guy to win in archery right? Oh yeah... Nick Vujicic has tetra-amelia syndrome, a condition characterized by the absence of arms and legs.

Nick would most likely win in archery over those who have both arms and legs without a blindfold and without self-confidence. Nick has overcome himself to the point that anything he decides to do, though others may say it's impossible, he will make it a possibility. This is the attitude needed to achieve your goal. You must have a vision of where you want to go or you won't like where you end up. When you make a goal, don't mistake it with a wish. A goal has a plan, a strategy, a method and principles. A wish is like living in America with a destination to go to Nigeria without a boat, a compass, a plan, or a passport. It's a GPS without the route and without the ETA.

So, first you need to have a target, know where your target is, know when you'll reach your target and then put a game plan together on how to hit that target. In order to hit that target, you must aim past that target, unless it's specific. Let's break this down:

- What is your target?
- Why is this your target?
- Where are you, compared to your target?
- How do you reach your target or reach through your target?
- Execute the game plan
- Enjoy the journey
- Reflect on the process

Write down what you want to achieve.

Give yourself permission to believe that you can achieve it and then believe it no matter what anyone else says.

Write down why you want to achieve this goal and what it means to you. Get deep and personal with this one.

Be honest with yourself and record where you currently are in that field of expertise - you'll want this to track your results later.

Determine if you need to reach a specific goal like a weight level or if it's an accomplishment you will be better off reaching beyond the target. Then map out step by step what it will take each day, week, month and/or year to reach your goal. Put a date on it.

Take action! Work work work.

This is a journey to a better you, so no matter the ups and downs, make sure you enjoy every moment of it. Remember that you are creating a wonderful life that is better than the most exciting movie you know!

After you've reached the date set, reflect on the lessons learned, the results you've gained and adjust your action level if you haven't reached your goal yet.

One of my mentors once said, "Most people stop right before reaching the next level." Don't be the one to stop. Push past your limiting beliefs like Master Roshi taught Goku and Krillin. Hold yourself accountable to your own training and remember that you learn and catch more value in battle than on the sidelines. And be willing to get alone, like Jack, to pay attention and reflect on what specific abilities you need to develop to reach your desired outcome. Be a part of the 20%.

Bonus

I'm going to share a secret with you about weight-lifting that not many recognize. This has, by the way, been recognized by the late great legendary Bruce Lee. As a matter of fact, one of his training methods helped me understand this truth. Here it is... All lifting weights is, is flexing your muscles. If you just flexed your muscles, depending on the intensity of the flex, you can reap the benefits of weight-training. The next time you go to lift weights, pay attention to what your muscles do when you lift. You'll see that they are flexing because of the resistance of the weight. You can create that same resistance on your own. Bruce Lee used to stand in the mirror and flex, release, then flex and repeat. How do you think he got the nickname Mr. Body? (K. Mckay, 2024; B. Mckay, 2024). Now he did eventually use actual weights later, and in my opinion, weight-training is a faster way to get results especially if your goal is to bulk up, but nevertheless, the effectiveness of this technique should not be underestimated.

You can contract your muscles at any time to create the resistance it takes to develop muscle. Try it the next time you're walking. Normally our gait is relaxed and rhythmic. This time when you walk, flex your feet muscle, your calf muscles and your tibialis anterior. It may feel weird at first, but you gain more body control the more you're aware of your ability to contract muscle and isolate muscle groups.

What other muscle groups can you use?

Have fun exploring and writing to me of your new discoveries and goals you plan to achieve. You can email me at the address provided below.

If you enjoyed this read, please take a moment to write a review. I'd love to see your feedback. I would love to hear from you!

Happy training.

As stated before, I'm a trainer with products.

If you've made it to the end, I'll give you **20% off** any product you choose; just email me with the subject: **"TRAIN"**

For info or inquiries about training or dietary supplements, contact me at:

antoniosavage7@gmail.com

Or scan this :

References

1. Heidelberger, M.: (n.d.). "Weight, There's More! The Risks and Benefits of Using Ankle and Wrist Weights" *SimpliFaster.*

   https://simplifaster.com/articles/ankle-wrist-weights-risks-benefits/

2. Helmstetter, S., & Schwartz, B. (1996). *Self-Talk for Weight Loss: Lose Weight, Keep It Off, and Never Diet Again.* St Martins Pr.

3. Ameridisability. (2018, October 24). "How Satoshi Tajiri, a Game Designer with Autism, Created an International Phenomenon" *Ameridisability.*

   https://www.ameridisability.com/satoshi-tajiri-how-a-little-known-game-designer-used-his-autism-to-create-an-international-phenomenon/#:~:text=by%20today%E2%80%94Pok%C3%A9mon.-,An%20international%20phenomenon,%E2%80%9Cthat's%20what%20Pok%C3%A9mon%20is.%E2%80%9D

4. MasterClass. (2021, August 16). "Walking With Weights Exercise: How to Walk With Weights Safely" *MasterClass.*

   https://www.masterclass.com/articles/walking-with-weights-guide

5. National Institutes of Health. (2011, July 11). *Zinc 'sparks' fly from egg within minutes of fertilization.*

   https://www.nih.gov/news-events/news-releases/zinc-sparks-fly-egg-within-minutes-fertilization

6. Vitamin. (n.d.). In *Wikipedia*. Retrieved October 14, 2024, from

    https://en.wikipedia.org/wiki/Vitamin#:~:text=Vitamins%20are%20organic%20molecule
    s%20(or,be%20obtained%20through%20the%20diet

7. Carpenter, K. , Weininger, . Jean , Truswell, . A. Stewart and Kent-Jones, . Douglas W.

    (2024, April 11). human nutrition. Encyclopedia Britannica.

    https://www.britannica.com/science/human-nutrition

8. National Research Council (1989). *Recommended Dietary Allowances* [E-publisher

    version]. https://nap.nationalacademies.org/read/1349/chapter/1

9. Lee SH, Moore LV, Park S, Harris DM, Blanck HM. "Adults Meeting Fruit and

    Vegetable Intake Recommendations — United States, 2019" (2022, January 7). *Morbidity

    and Mortality Weekly Report*. http://dx.doi.org/10.15585/mmwr.mm7101a1

10. National Sanitation Foundation. (n.d.). *Supplement and Vitamin Certification*.

    https://www.nsf.org/consumer-resources/articles/supplement-vitamin-certification

11. Mayo Clinic. (n.d.). *Nutrition for kids: Guidelines for a healthy diet*.

    https://www.mayoclinic.org/healthy-lifestyle/childrens-health/in-depth/nutrition-for-kids/
    art-20049335

12. Kern, C. (2023, May 10). *Why antibiotics aren't always the answer for an illness*. MAYO

    CLINIC HEALTH SYSTEM.

    https://www.mayoclinichealthsystem.org/hometown-health/speaking-of-health/3-reasons-
    why-you-did-not-receive-antibiotics-from-your-provider

13. Hu, L., Ji, J., Li, D., Meng, J., & Yu, B. (2021). The combined effect of vitamin K and

    calcium on bone mineral density in humans: a meta-analysis of randomized controlled trials. *Journal of orthopaedic surgery and research, 16*(1), 592.

https://doi.org/10.1186/s13018-021-02728-4

14. U.S. Food & Drug Administration. (2023, May 16). *Facts about Dietary Supplements.*

https://www.fda.gov/news-events/rumor-control/facts-about-dietary-supplements#:~:text
=More%20Information:%20The%20FDA%20does,too%20good%20to%20be%20true

15. Casagrande Tango R. (2003). Psychiatric side effects of medications prescribed in

internal medicine. *Dialogues in clinical neuroscience, 5*(2), 155–165.

https://doi.org/10.31887/DCNS.2003.5.2/rcasagrandetango

16. Mckay, K., & Mckay, B. (2024, July 25). *The Secrets to Bruce Lee's Legendary Physical*

Training. ART OF MANLINESS.

https://www.artofmanliness.com/health-fitness/fitness/bruce-lee-workout/

Acknowledgement

First and foremost I would like to thank my wife Priscilla for helping me put the finishing touches on editing, and for being a big motivation, an example, and a supporter in writing this book. You help me to be better every day.

I want to acknowledge Akira Toriyama for the memories and lessons that will live with me forever. May your family be blessed and your legacy live on.

I want to thank Satoshi Tajiri - the creator of Pokémon - for making learning fun and interesting. The lessons I learned from your contribution to the world have helped me in numerous ways in my life journey.

I want to thank Genndy Tartakovsky for creating such a cool American anime. I always looked forward to watching the next episode of Samurai Jack and seeing how he would better himself to overcome the next obstacle. I learned to do that.

I want to thank my Capoeira Mestre, Mestre Preto Velho. You trained my body as well as my mind with the philosophy that I still live by today and prepared me for my future. Thank you.